Diabetic Air Fryer Cookbook for Beginners

Healthy and Easy Air Fryer Recipes

To Prevent and Control Diabetes

Lilith Ballard

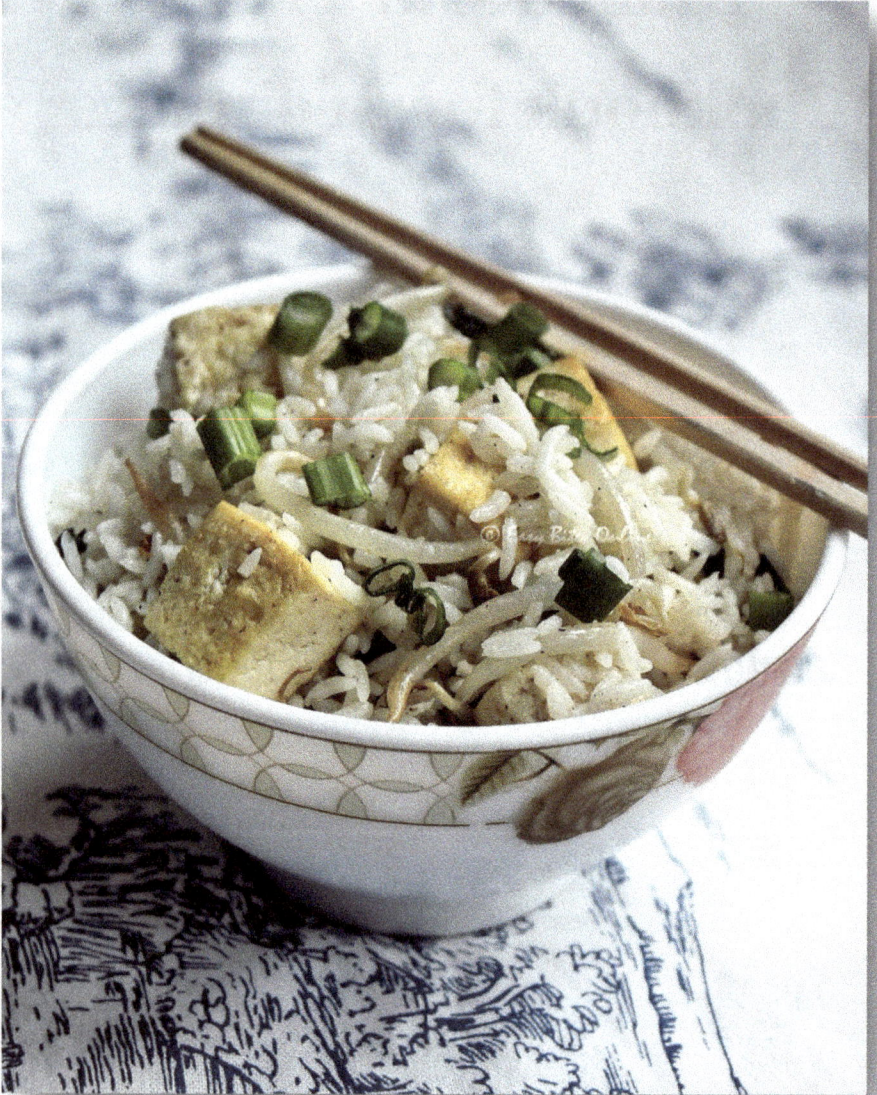

Table of Contents

APPLE CHIPS

Preparation Time: 6 minutes

Cooking Time: 18 minutes

Servings: 4

Nutritional values:

- Calories: 104 kcal
- Fat: 3 g
- Carbohydrates: 2 g
- Proteins: 1 g

Ingredients:

- Cooking spray
- 2 tsp. canola oil
- ¼ cup plain low-fat Greek yogurt
- 1 tsp. honey
- 1 tsp. ground cinnamon

- 1 tbsp. almond butter
- 1 apple

Directions:

1. Slice the apple into thin slices.
2. Mix the slices of apple with oil and cinnamon before you toss them together for even coating.
3. Apply cooking spray on your air fryer basket.
4. Place the slices of apple in the air fryer basket. Don't place more than 8 slices on a single layer.
5. Cook the apple at 375°F for 12 minutes. Ensure you rearrange the slices of apple after every 4 minutes. It is possible that the apple chips are not crispy enough when you remove them from your air fryer. They will become even crispier as they cool.
6. If there are slices of apple left, you can do the same thing to them.
7. Mix the honey, almond butter, and yogurt together evenly. Add a dollop of the sauce to every serving of the apple chips.

VEGGIE QUESADILLAS

Preparation Time: 21 minutes

Cooking Time: 18 minutes

Servings: 4

Nutritional values:

- Calories: 291 kcal
- Fat: 8 g
- Carbohydrates: 12 g
- Proteins: 17 g

Ingredients:

- Cooking spray
- 4 sprouted whole-grain flour tortillas
- 4 ounces reduced-fat sharp Cheddar cheese, shredded (about 1 cup)
- 2 tbsp. chopped fresh cilantro
- 2 ounces plain reduced-fat Greek yogurt
- ¼ tsp. ground cumin
- ½ cup drained refrigerated Pico de gallo

- 1 tsp. lime zest plus 1 tbsp. fresh juice (from 1 lime)
- 1 cup sliced zucchini
- 1 cup sliced red bell pepper
- 1 cup no-salt-added canned black beans, drained, and rinsed

Directions:

1. Sprinkle 2 tbsp. of shredded cheese over half of each tortilla. After that, you can add cheese on the tortilla. Also, add black beans, slices of zucchini, and a quarter cup of red pepper slices on the tortilla as well.

2. Sprinkle the remaining cheese on the tortilla. Now, you can fold the tortilla in the shape of half-moon. They will now become quesadillas. We hope you understand that quesadillas are tortillas with fillings.

3. Coat the quesadillas with cooking spray and secure them with toothpicks.

4. Coat the air fryer basket with cooking spray. Then, you can place the quesadillas in the basket. Cook them at 400°F until they turn golden brown and crispy. This should happen after about 10 minutes of cooking. Remember to turn the quesadillas over after 5 minutes. You can air fry all the quesadillas at once or in two batches.

5. While the quesadillas are being cooked, mix the cumin, lime juice, lime zest, and yogurt together in a bowl.

6.   You need to cut each of the quesadillas into wedges before you serve them. It is also necessary to sprinkle cilantro on them. Serve each of them with a tbsp. of cumin and 2 tbsp. of Pico de Gallo

GREEK FETA FRIES

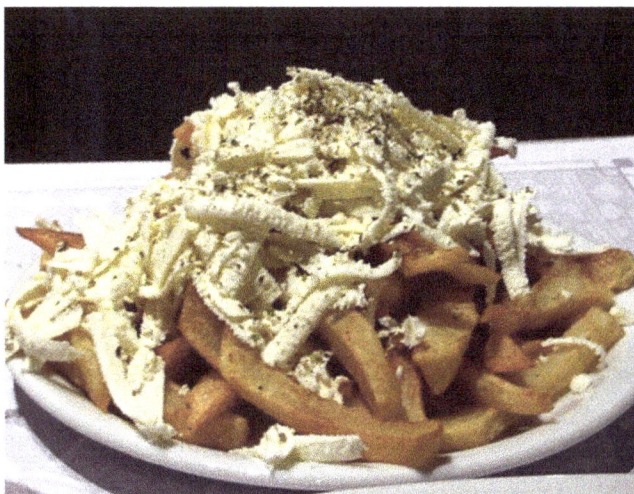

Preparation Time: 12 minutes

Cooking Time: 15-20 minutes

Servings: 2

Nutritional values:

- Calories: 383 kcal
- Fat: 16 g
- Carbohydrates: 20 g
- Proteins: 19 g

Ingredients:

- Cooking spray
- 2 potatoes, scrubbed and dried
- 1 tbsp. olive oil
- 2 tsp. lemon zest
- ½ tsp. dried oregano
- ¼ tsp. kosher salt
- ¼ tsp. garlic powder
- ¼ tsp. onion powder
- ¼ tsp. paprika
- ¼ tsp. black pepper
- 2 ounces feta cheese, finely grated (about ½ cup)
- 2 ounces shredded skinless rotisserie chicken breast
- ¼ cup prepared tzatziki
- ¼ cup seeded and diced plum tomato
- 2 tbsp. chopped red onion
- 1 tbsp. chopped fresh flat-leaf parsley and oregano

Directions:

1. Preheat an air fryer to 380°F. Coat the basket with cooking spray. Now, you should cut each potato into ¼-inch thick slices.

2. Mix the potatoes together with some oil. Add the pepper, paprika, onion powder, garlic powder, salt, and dried

oregano together with zest. Season the potatoes with the zest mixture.

3. Air fry the potatoes for about 7 minutes. Turn them over and cook them for another 8 minutes. The potatoes should be crispy by then.

4. Remove the potato fries and top it with herbs, red onion, tomato, remaining feta, chicken, and tzatziki. You can now serve the meal.

ROASTED VEGETABLES

Preparation Time: 5 minutes

Cooking Time: 18 minutes

Servings: 4

Nutritional values:

- Calories: 81 kcal
- Fat: 4 g
- Carbohydrates: 8 g
- Proteins: 3 g

Ingredients:

- ¼ cup parmesan cheese
- ¼ cup balsamic vinegar
- ½ cup yellow squash, sliced
- ½ cup sliced mushrooms
- ½ cup baby zucchini, sliced
- ½ cup baby carrots
- 1 tsp. sea salt
- 1 tsp. red pepper flakes

- 1 tsp. black pepper
- 1 tbsp. olive oil
- 1 tbsp. minced garlic
- 1 small onion, sliced
- 1 cup cauliflower florets
- 1 cup broccoli florets

Directions:

1. The first step is to preheat your air fryer at 400°F for 3 minutes. Now, add red pepper flakes, pepper, salt, garlic, balsamic vinegar, and olive oil together in a bowl. Whisk them together until they mix up evenly.
2. Add vegetables to the mixture and toss them together.
3. Put the vegetables in your air fryer basket and cook it for 6 minutes.
4. Shake it and cook for another 6 to 8 minutes.
5. Add some cheese to it before you cook it for another 2 minutes.
6. By now, it should be ready for consumption.

CRISPY PORK BELLY CRACK

Preparation Time: 5 minutes

Cooking Time: 25 minutes

Servings: 4

Nutritional values:

- Calories: 332 kcal
- Fat: 24 g
- Carbohydrates: 20 g
- Proteins: 26 g

Ingredients:

- ½ tsp. pepper
- 1 tsp. sea salt
- 1 lb. raw pork belly strips

Directions:

1. Start by slicing the pork belly strips. The idea is to cut the pork into sizes that can be chewed easily.

2. Mix the salt and pepper tighter evenly in a small bowl.

3. Put the pieces of pork belly in the mixture and toss them for even coating.

4. Preheat your air fryer for about 3 minutes

5. Now, put the pieces of pork in your air fryer basket.

6. Set the temperature to about 390°F and cook the pork for about 15 minutes, but make sure you turn them over every 5 minutes.

7. After 15 minutes, they should be crispy and done.

8. Sometimes, they may take a little longer, or they could take less than 15 minutes. That's why you need to keep checking them every 5 minutes.

9. Drain them on paper towels. Now, you can serve them either hot or warm. Enjoy your tasty meal. You can add more spices to yours. Cooking requires being creative.

CRISPY GARLIC KETO CROUTONS

Preparation Time: 12 minutes

Cooking Time: 10 minutes

Servings: 1

Nutritional values:

- Calories: 50 kcal
- Fat: 4 g
- Carbohydrates: 1 g
- Proteins: 2 g

Ingredients:

- 2 tbsp. Olive Oil
- 2 Cups Keto Farmers Bread or half of the loaf
- ½ tbsp. garlic powder
- 1 tbsp. Marjoram

Directions:

1. Cut your bread into several slices and cut each slice into smaller squares.

2. Place the pieces of bread into a bowl and add the other three ingredients to it. Mix them together.

3. Now, pour the croutons mixture into your air fryer basket. Make sure everything is on a single layer for crispiness. Don't add additional oil. An air fryer works best with little oil.

4. Air fry the bread for about 10 minutes to make it crispy. However, you need to shake it after 5 minutes. We suggest you select medium to high heat.

5. After about 10 minutes, the croutons should be ready for consumption.

6. Remove the croutons and give them 5 minutes to cool down before you serve them.

7. Enjoy the recipe!

TOMATOES AND CHEESE FRITTATA

Preparation Time: 7 minutes

Cooking Time: 10 minutes

Servings: 4

Nutritional values:

- Calories: 186
- Fat: 11.1 g
- Carbohydrates: 9.1 g
- Proteins: 11.9 g

Ingredients:

- 8 eggs
- 2 tomatoes
- ¼ cup milk, fat-free
- ½ cup cheddar cheese, reduced-fat
- 2 leeks, sliced

- 1 tbsp. fresh thyme
- Pinch salt
- Pinch pepper

Directions:

1. Preheat the Air Fryer to 330°F.
2. In a baking dish, grease leeks with olive oil. Add eggs, cheese, salt, and pepper. Layer tomato slices on top.
3. Place baking dish onside the Air fryer basket. Cook for 10 minutes.
4. Remove and transfer the frittata to a plate. Sprinkle with thyme. Serve.

EGG WHITE AND FLAX CREPES

Preparation Time: 8 minutes

Cooking Time: 26 minutes

Servings: 3

Nutritional values:

- Calories: 78.7
- Fat: 5.3 g
- Carbohydrates: 5.5 g
- Proteins: 3.1 g

Ingredients:

- 3 egg whites only
- 2 tbsp. ground flaxseed
- 2 eggs
- ¼ cup coconut flour
- ¼ cup almond milk
- ½ tsp. baking soda

Directions:

1. Combine all ingredients in a food processor or blender and blend until thoroughly combined.

2. Pour batter into the air fryer hot skillet covered with cooking spray and swirl around to create a large, thin circle.

3. Let cook until bubbles in the batter begin to pop, gently easing up the sides every few moments, about 3 minutes or less.

4. Flip crepes and cook on the other side until firm. Serve.

SCRAMBLED TOFU

Preparation Time: 7 minutes

Cooking Time: 10-12 minutes

Servings: 2

Nutritional values:

- Calories: 100
- Fat: 5 g
- Carbohydrates: 6 g
- Proteins: 8 g

Ingredients:

- 4-6 whole wheat tortillas, warmed
- 2 14-ounce blocks extra-firm tofu
- 1 15-ounce can black beans, rinsed, drained
- 2 tbsp. vegetable oil
- 1 onion, chopped
- ½ tsp. ground cumin
- ½ tsp. ground coriander
- 1 green bell pepper, chopped finely

- 1 red bell pepper, chopped finely
- 1 ½ tsp. ground turmeric
- ¼ cup coarsely chopped fresh cilantro
- Salt
- Ground pepper

Garnishes:

- Salsa
- scallions, sliced
- Cheddar, grated
- Avocado, chopped

Directions:

1. Place tofu on a plate lined with several layers of paper towels. Smash tofu using a fork or potato masher.
2. Put onion and peppers in the Air fryer basket. Cook for 2 minutes. Season with cumin and coriander. Cook for 1 minute.
3. Add in tofu. Stir in turmeric. Add beans; cook, often stirring, until heated through, 1–2 minutes. Stir in cilantro; season with salt and pepper.
4. Serve scrambled with tortillas and garnishes, as desired.

BELL PEPPER, SALSA, AND TACO FRITTATA

Preparation Time: 11 minutes

Cooking Time: 24 minutes

Servings: 4

Nutritional values:

- Calories: 140
- Fat: 17 g
- Carbohydrates: 5.3 g
- Proteins: 17.6 g

Ingredients:

- 6 eggs
- ¾ cup cheddar cheese, reduced-fat
- ¼ cup onions, chopped
- ¼ cup green bell peppers, chopped
- 1 cup salsa
- 2 tbsp. taco seasoning

- 1 cup sour cream, low fat
- 1 oz. milk, low fat
- Pinch salt
- Pinch pepper

Directions:

1. Preheat USA Air Fryer to 330°F.
2. Combine eggs, green bell pepper, taco seasoning, onions, milk, cheddar cheese, salt, and pepper in a bowl.
3. Transfer mixture to a baking dish. Lightly grease with cooking spray. Put baking dish inside the Air Fryer basket. Cook for 20 minutes.
4. Top with salsa and sour cream. Serve.

SPINACH WITH TOMATO SALSA FRITTATA

Preparation Time: 9 minutes

Cooking Time: 10 minutes

Servings: 3

Nutritional values:

- Calories: 180
- Fat: 24.1 g
- Carbohydrates: 5.73 g
- Proteins: 14.3 g

Ingredients:

For the frittata:

- 1 package spinach
- 1 tbsp. extra-virgin olive oil
- 2 cloves garlic, minced
- 1 small onion, sliced
- 1 cup applesauce

- 1/3 cup coconut milk
- ½ cup Tofutti cheese

For the salsa:

- 4 plum tomatoes, chopped
- 2 scallions, minced
- 2 tbsp. fresh cilantro minced
- 1 tbsp. lime juice
- 1 clove garlic, minced
- ¼ tsp. salt
- 1/8 tsp. pepper

Directions:

1. Preheat the Air Fryer to 350°F.
2. Add the garlic and onion and cook, stirring, for 3 minutes or until translucent. Toss in the spinach. Transfer to a dish. Set aside.
3. Meanwhile, in a large bowl, pour the applesauce and milk. Whisk until frothy.
4. Pour applesauce mixture into a baking dish. Place garlic, onion, and spinach.
5. Transfer to the Air Fryer and cook for 7 minutes. Sprinkle with cheese. Serve.

BREADED SQUASH BLOOMS

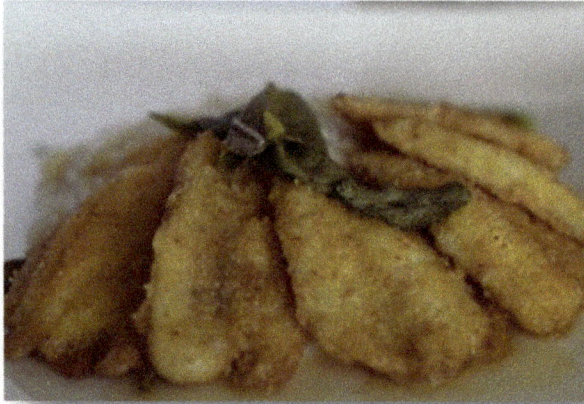

Preparation Time: 10 minutes

Cooking Time: 24 minutes

Servings: 3

Nutritional values:

- Calories: 5
- Fat: 0.2 g
- Carbohydrates: 1 g
- Proteins: 0.1 g

Ingredients:

- 2½ pounds squash flowers, rinsed
- 1 cup coconut flour, finely milled
- Pinch sea salt, to taste
- raisin vinegar for garnish, optional

Directions:

1. Preheat Air Fryer to 330°F.
2. Season squash blossoms with salt. Dredge into coconut flour.
3. Layer breaded blossoms in the air fryer basket. Fry for 2 minutes or until golden brown. Drain on paper towels.
4. Stack cooked squash blossoms in the middle of plates. Sprinkle raisin vinegar. Serve.

STUFFED ZUCCHINI FLOWERS

Preparation Time: 11 minutes

Cooking Time: 5-10 minutes

Servings: 3

Nutritional values:

- Calories: 5
- Fat: 0 g
- Carbohydrates: 1 g
- Proteins: 0 g

Ingredients:

- 20 zucchini flowers

Filling:

- 2 tsp. sour cream, reduce fat
- ¼ cup cream cheese, reduced-fat
- ½ cup goat cheese, reduced-fat

- 2 tsp. fresh basil leaves, minced
- 1/8 cup fresh chives, minced
- Pinch black pepper

Batter:

- 1½ cups sparkling water, sugar-free
- 1½ cups coconut flour, finely milled
- 1 tsp. sea salt

Directions:

1. Preheat Air Fryer to 330°F.
2. In a bowl, combine sour cream, cream cheese, goat cheese, basil leaves, chives, and pepper.
3. Spoon equal portions into zucchini flowers. Twist flower tips for sealing. Set aside and freeze until ready to fry.
4. Mix water, coconut flour, and salt in a bowl. Mix until well combined. Dip stuffed zucchini flower.
5. Slide stuffed flowers into the air fryer basket. Fry until lightly browned. Drain on paper towels. Serve.

AIR FRYER BISCUITS

Preparation Time: 12 minutes

Cooking Time: 13 minutes

Servings: 8

Nutritional values:

- Calories :151 kcal
- Fat: 7 g
- Carbohydrates: 16 g
- Proteins: 6 g

Ingredients:

- 175 grams self-rising flour
- 1 tsp. mustard powder
- 1 tbsp. thyme
- Pinch salt
- Dash pepper
- 25 grams butter

- 75 grams grated cheddar cheese
- 1 medium egg
- 30 ml whole milk

Directions:

1. Combine in a large mixing bowl the butter, flour, mustard powder, thyme, salt, and pepper.
2. With your hands, rub the fat into the flour mixture to form into coarse breadcrumbs.
3. Add in the whole milk, egg, and cheese to the flour mixture, mix with a fork and then finally mix it with your hands to form a large biscuit dough ball.
4. Dust your work surface with a little flour.
5. Roll out the dough ball with a rolling pin. Using biscuit cutters, form the dough into biscuit rounds.
6. Arrange the biscuit rounds in the air fryer grill pan at least 1 inch apart as they grow during cooking.
7. Cook the biscuits for 8 minutes at 360°F. Serve hot over the stew.

AIR FRYER MASHED POTATO CAKES

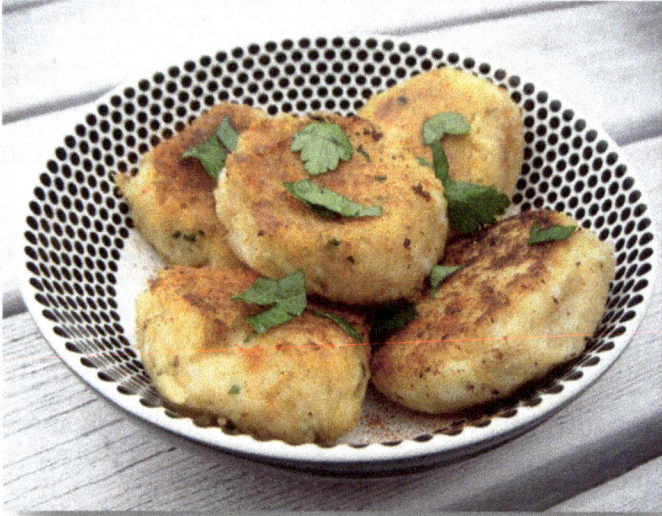

Preparation Time: 6 minutes

Cooking Time: 24 minutes

Servings: 12

Nutritional values:

- Calories :207 kcal
- Fat: 8 g

- Carbohydrates: 23 g
- Proteins: 7 g

Ingredients:

- 6 to 8 strips cooked and crumbled bacon
- 2 cups mashed potatoes
- ¼ cup g diced green onion
- 1 cup shredded cheddar cheese
- ½ tsp. pepper
- 1 tsp. salt
- 2 beaten eggs
- 2 cups panko crumbs
- 1 cup flour

Directions:

1. Place the bacon in a skillet on medium heat; fry until crispy. Drain bacon on a plate lined with a paper towel.
2. When cooled, crumble the bacon into small bits and transfer to a large bowl.
3. Add the mashed potatoes, green onions, and cheddar cheese to the bowl, stirring to combine well.
4. Prepare a baking pan by lining it with parchment paper.

5.   Scrape the mashed potato mixture into the baking pan and evenly spread up to the sides. Freeze for half an hour to solidify. Remove from freezer.

6.   With a round cookie cutter, cut circles out of the potato mixture, set aside, and then continue cutting out the circles.

7.   Pour the flour in a bowl, and then the beaten eggs in a small bowl, and the panko breadcrumbs in another bowl.

8.   Start dipping the potato cake flour in the bowl with flour.

9.   Dip in the bowl with beaten eggs and dredge in the panko crumbs, making sure that it is well coated.

10.   Load the potato cake into the air fryer in a single layer.

11.   Cook the potato cake for 7 to 9 minutes at 370°F.

12.   Serve crispy and hot.

AIR FRYER BANANA BREAD

Preparation Time: 8 minutes

Cooking Time: 30-35 minutes

Servings: 8

Nutritional values:

- Calories :180 kcal
- Fat: 6 g
- Carbohydrates: 29 g
- Proteins: 4 g

Ingredients:

- 3/4 cup white-whole wheat flour
- ¼ tsp. baking soda
- ½ tsp. kosher salt
- 1 tsp. cinnamon
- 2 lightly beaten large eggs
- 2 medium mashed ripe bananas (yield 3/4 cup)
- 1 tsp. vanilla extract
- 1/3 cup plain nonfat yogurt

- 2 tbsp. vegetable oil
- ½ cup granulated sugar
- 2 tbsp. roughly chopped toasted walnuts
- Cooking spray

Directions:

1. Prepare a six-inch round cake pan and line the bottom with a parchment paper; lightly grease with cooking spray.
2. Whisk in a medium-sized bowl the flour, baking soda, cinnamon, and salt. Set aside.
3. Whisk in a separate bowl the eggs, mashed bananas, yogurt, sugar, vanilla, and oil.
4. Slowly fold the banana mixture into the flour mixture until incorporated.
5. Pour the batter into the cake pan and spread on top with walnuts. Heat a 5.3-quart air fryer at 310°F.
6. Place the cake pan in the heated air fryer and cook the batter for thirty to thirty-five minutes until done. Turn the pan halfway through cooking time.
7. Place the pan on a wire rack and let cool for fifteen minutes before removing and slicing.
8. Serve!

AIR FRYER CHURROS WITH CHOCOLATE SAUCE

Preparation Time: 6 minutes

Cooking Time: 27 minutes

Servings: 12

Nutritional values:

- Calories :173 kcal
- Fat: 11 g
- Carbohydrates: 12 g
- Proteins: 3 g

Ingredients:

- ½ cup water
- ¼ cup, plus 2 tbsp. unsalted butter, divided
- ¼ tsp. kosher salt
- 2 large eggs
- ½ cup all-purpose flour
- 2 tsp. ground cinnamon

- 1/3 cup granulated sugar
- 3 tbsp. heavy cream
- 4 ounces finely chopped bittersweet baking chocolate
- 2 tbsp. vanilla kefir

Directions:

1. In a small saucepan, bring ¼ cup of butter, salt, and water to a boil on medium-high heat.

2. Stir in flour vigorously using a wooden spoon form thirty seconds on medium-low heat.

3. Stir and cook for 2 to 3 minutes until the dough starts to detach from the sides of the saucepan and film formation is beginning to develop on the bottom of your pan.

4. Place the dough in a medium-size bowl, frequently stirring, for 1 minute until slightly cooled.

5. Add the eggs to the dough one at a time, often stirring, until the mixture is smooth.

6. Pour the mixture into a piping bag attached with a medium-sized star tip. Refrigerate for half an hour.

7. Pipe about six pieces with a length of 3 inches in an air fryer basket; make sure to arrange them in a single layer.

8. Cook the batter at 380°F for ten minutes until nicely golden. Do the rest of the remaining batter. In a medium bowl, mix the cinnamon and sugar.

9. Brush the cooked churros with 2 tbsp. of melted butter; roll churros in sugar mixture until well coated.

10. Put together in a small microwave-proof bowl the bittersweet baking chocolate and heavy cream. Microwave the mixture for 30 seconds on high until smooth and melted. Stir after fifteen seconds and add the kefir.

11. Serve with chocolate sauce.

AIR FRYER STRAWBERRY POP-TARTS

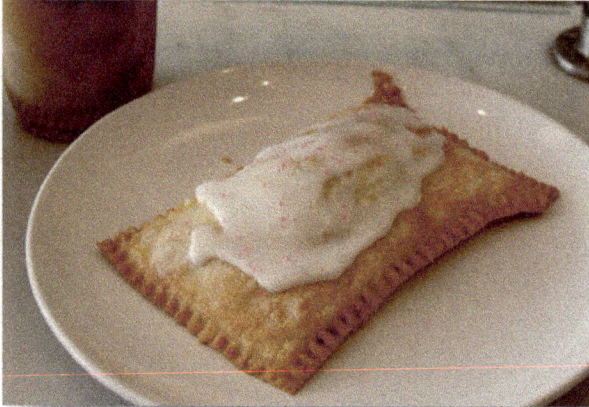

Preparation Time: 12 minutes

Cooking Time: 22 minutes

Servings: 6

Nutritional values:

- Calories: 229 kcal
- Fat: 9 g
- Carbohydrates: 39 g
- Proteins: 2 g

Ingredients:

- ¼ cup granulated sugar
- 8 ounces quartered strawberries
- ½ (14.1 ounces) package refrigerated piecrusts
- Cooking spray
- 1 ½ tsp. fresh lemon juice from 1 lemon
- ½ cup powdered sugar
- ½ ounce rainbow candy sprinkles

Directions:

1. In a medium-size heatproof bowl, stir granulated sugar and strawberries until well coated. Let strawberry stand for 15 minutes, stirring often.

2. Microwave the sugarcoated strawberries on high for ten minutes until glossy and shrunk. Stir mixture halfway throughout cooking, let cool for half an hour.

3. Prepare the pie crust and roll into a twelve-inch circle on a surface lightly dusted with flour.

4. Cut the dough into 12 rectangular pieces, about 2 ½"by3" and reroll the scraps.

5. Fill the center of six of the rectangular pieces with two tsp. of strawberry mixture. Leave at least half-inch allowance on the border.

6.　　Brush the edges of dough rectangles with water and cover the filling with another piece of the dough rectangle. Press the edges of the dough with fork tines to seal completely. Coat the tarts with cooking spray.

7.　　Place three pieces of tarts in a single layer of your air fryer basket. Cook for ten minutes at 350°F until golden brown.

8.　　Repeat the same steps for the rest of the tart. Let cool on a wire rack for half an hour.

9.　　Prepare the glaze by stirring the sugar in lemon juice until smooth and spoon into cooled tarts.

10.　　Evenly sprinkle on top with candy sprinkles.

11.　　Serve!

AIR-FRIED PEACH HAND PIES

Preparation Time: 11 minutes

Cooking Time: 26 minutes

Servings: 8

Nutritional values:

- Calories: 314 kcal
- Fat: 16 g
- Carbohydrates: 43 g
- Proteins: 3 g

Ingredients:

- 2 (5 ounces) peeled and chopped fresh peaches
- 3 tbsp. granulated sugar
- 1 tbsp. fresh lemon juice from 1 lemon
- ¼ tsp. table salt
- 1 tsp. vanilla extract
- 1 tsp. cornstarch

- 1 (14.1 ounces) package refrigerated piecrusts
- Cooking spray

Directions:

1. Mix together in a medium bowl the peaches, sugar, lemon juice, salt, and vanilla, often stir, and let stand for fifteen minutes.

2. Drain the peaches in a colander; reserve one tbsp. of soaking liquid.

3. Whisk the cornstarch into the liquid and then add to the drained peaches.

4. Cut the pie crust into eight 4" circles.

5. Fill the center of crust circles with 1 tbsp. each of peaches filling; crimping the edges with fork tines to seal.

6. Cut three small slits on the top of hand pies. Coat the pies with a liberal amount of cooking spray.

7. Arrange three-hand pies in a single layer of your air fryer basket. Cook at 350°F for 12 to 14 minutes until golden brown. Cook the rest of the hand pies.

FLAVORED PORK CHOPS

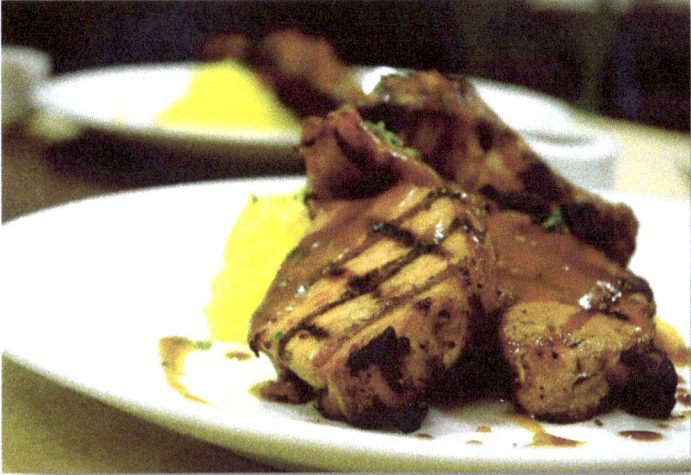

Preparation Time: 9 minutes

Cooking Time: 38 minutes

Servings: 2

Nutritional values:

- Calories: 118 kcal
- Fat: 3.41 g
- Carbohydrates: 0 g
- Proteins: 22 g

Ingredients:

- 3 cloves ground garlic
- 2 tbsp. olive oil
- 1 tbsp. marinade
- 4 thawed pork chops

Directions:

1. Mix the cloves of ground garlic, marinade, and oil. Then apply this mixture on the chops.
2. Put the chops in the air fryer at 360°F for 35 minutes.

POTATOES WITH LOIN AND CHEESE

Preparation Time: 5 minutes

Cooking Time: 32 minutes

Servings: 4

Nutritional values:

- Calories: 382 kcal
- Fat: 3.41 g
- Carbohydrates: 2 g
- Proteins: 2.9 g

Ingredients:

- 1kg potatoes
- 1 large onion
- 1 piece roasted loin
- Extra virgin olive oil
- Salt

- Ground pepper
- Grated cheese

Directions:

1. Peel the potatoes, cut the cane, wash, and dry.
2. Put salt and add some threads of oil; we bind well.
3. Pass the potatoes to the basket of the air fryer and select 180°C, 20 minutes.
4. Meanwhile, in a pan, put some extra virgin olive oil, add the peeled onion, and cut it into julienne.
5. When the onion is transparent, add the chopped loin.
6. Sauté well and pepper.
7. Put the potatoes on a baking sheet.
8. Add the onion with the loin.
9. Cover with a layer of grated cheese.
10. Bake a little until the cheese takes heat and melts.

SPICED PORK CHOPS

Preparation Time: 8 minutes

Cooking Time: 11 minutes

Servings: 2

Nutritional values:

- Calories: 118 kcal
- Fat: 6.85 g
- Carbohydrates: 0.3 g
- Proteins: 13.12 g

Ingredients:

- 2 boneless pork chops
- 15 ml vegetable oil
- 25 g dark brown sugar, packaged
- 6 g Hungarian paprika
- 2 g ground mustard
- 2 g freshly ground black pepper
- 3 g onion powder

- 3 g garlic powder
- Salt and pepper to taste

Directions:

1. Preheat the air fryer for a few minutes at 180°C.
2. Cover the pork chops with oil.
3. Put all the spices and season the pork chops abundantly, almost as if you were making them breaded.
4. Place the pork chops in the preheated air fryer.
5. Select Steak and set the time to 10 minutes.
6. Remove the pork chops when it has finished cooking. Let it stand for 5 minutes and serve.

PORK RIND

Preparation Time: 9 minutes

Cooking Time: 62 minutes

Servings: 4

Nutritional values:

- Calories: 282 kcal
- Fat: 23.41 g
- Carbohydrates: 0.3 g
- Proteins: 16.59 g

Ingredients:

- 1kg pork rinds
- Salt
- ½ tsp. black pepper coffee

Directions:

1. Preheat the air fryer. Set the time of 5 minutes and the temperature to 200°C.

2. Cut the bacon into cubes—1 finger wide.

3. Season with salt and a pinch of pepper.

4. Place in the basket of the air fryer. Set the time of 45 minutes and press the power button.

5. Shake the basket every 10 minutes so that the pork rinds stay golden brown equally.

6. Once they are ready, drain a little on the paper towel, so they stay dry. Transfer to a plate and serve.

MEATLOAF REBOOT

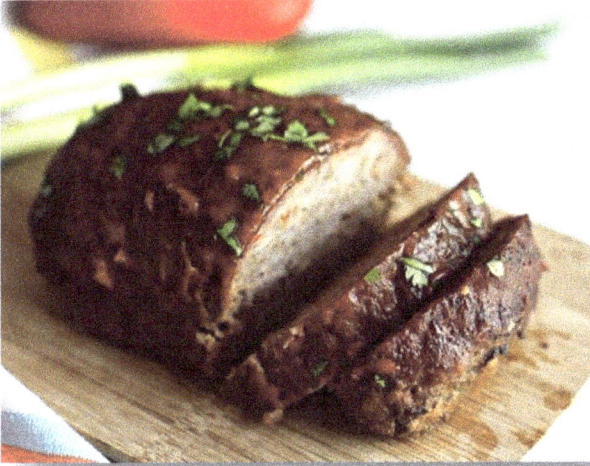

Preparation Time: 13 minutes

Cooking Time: 10-15 minutes

Servings: 2

Nutritional values:

- Calories: 201 kcal
- Fat: 5 g
- Carbohydrates: 9.6 g
- Proteins: 38 g

Ingredients:

- 4 slices leftover meatloaf, cut about 1-inch thick.

Directions:

1. Preheat your air fryer to 350°F.
2. Spray each side of the meatloaf slices with cooking spray. Add the slices to the air fryer and cook for about 9 to 10 minutes.
3. Don't turn the slices halfway through the cooking cycle because they may break apart. Instead, keep them on one side to cook to ensure they stay together

MEDITERRANEAN LAMB MEATBALLS

Preparation Time: 5 minutes

Cooking Time: 42 minutes

Servings: 4

Nutritional values:

- Calories: 282 kcal
- Fat: 23.41 g
- Carbohydrates: 0.1 g
- Proteins: 16.59 g

Ingredients:

- 454 g ground lamb
- 3 cloves garlic, minced
- 5 g salt
- 1 g black pepper
- 2 g mint, freshly chopped
- 2 g ground cumin

- 3 ml hot sauce
- 1 g chili powder
- 1 scallion, chopped
- 8 g parsley, finely chopped
- 15 ml fresh lemon juice
- 2 g lemon zest
- 10 ml olive oil

Directions:

1. Mix the lamb, garlic, salt, pepper, mint, cumin, hot sauce, chili powder, chives, parsley, lemon juice, and lemon zest until well combined.
2. Create balls with the lamb mixture and cool for 30 minutes.
3. Select Preheat in the air fryer and press Start/Pause.
4. Cover the meatballs with olive oil and place them in the preheated fryer.
5. Select Steak, set the time to 10 minutes, and press Start/Pause.

POTATOES WITH BACON, ONION, AND CHEESE

Preparation Time: 6 minutes

Cooking Time: 20-25 minutes

Servings: 4

Nutritional values:

- Calories: 120 kcal
- Fat: 3.41 g
- Carbohydrates: 1 g
- Proteins: 20.99 g

Ingredients:

- 200 g potatoes
- 150 g bacon
- 1 onion
- Slices of cheese
- Extra virgin olive oil
- Salt

Directions:

1. Peel the potatoes, cut into thin slices, and wash them well.

2. Drain and dry the potatoes, put salt and a few strands of extra virgin olive oil.

3. Stir well and place in the basket of the air fryer.

4. Cut the onion into julienne, put a little oil, and stir, place on the potatoes.

5. Finally, put the sliced bacon on the onion.

6. Take the basket to the air fryer and select 20 minutes, 180°C.

7. From time to time, remove the basket.

8. Take all the contents of the basket to a source and when it is still hot, place the slices of cheese on top.

9. You can let the heat of the potatoes melt the cheese, or you can gratin a few minutes in the oven.

PARMESAN GARLIC CRUSTED SALMON

Preparation Time: 5 minutes

Cooking Time: 18 minutes

Servings: 2

Nutritional values:

- Calories: 330 kcal
- Fat: 19 g
- Carbohydrates: 11 g
- Proteins: 31 g

Ingredients:

- Whole wheat breadcrumbs: ¼ cup
- 4 cups salmon
- 2 tbsp. butter, melted
- ¼ tsp. freshly ground black pepper
- ¼ cup Parmesan cheese (grated)

- 2 tsp. minced garlic
- ½ tsp. Italian seasoning

Directions:

- Pat dry the salmon. In a bowl, mix Parmesan cheese, Italian seasoning, and breadcrumbs. In another pan, mix melted butter with garlic and add to the breadcrumbs mix. Mix well
- Add kosher salt and freshly ground black pepper to salmon. On top of every salmon piece, add the crust mix and press gently.
- Preheat let the air fryer to 400°F, spray the oil over the air fryer basket.
- Cook salmon until done to your liking.
- Serve hot with vegetable side dishes.

AIR FRYER SALMON WITH MAPLE SOY GLAZE

Preparation Time: 5 minutes

Cooking Time: 8 minutes

Servings: 4

Nutritional values:

- Calories: 292 kcal
- Fat: 11 g
- Carbohydrates: 12 g
- Proteins: 35 g

Ingredients:

- 3 tbsp. pure maple syrup
- 3 tbsp. gluten-free soy sauce
- 1 tbsp. sriracha hot sauce
- 1 garlic clove, minced
- 4 salmon fillets, skinless

Directions:

1. In a Ziplock bag, mix sriracha, maple syrup, garlic, and soy sauce with salmon.
2. Mix well and let it marinate for at least half an hour.
3. Let the air fryer preheat to 400°F with oil spray the basket
4. Take fish out from the marinade, pat dry.
5. Put the salmon in the air fryer, cook for 7 to 8 minutes or longer.
6. In the meantime, in a saucepan, add the marinade, let it simmer until reduced to half.
7. Add glaze over salmon and serve.

AIR FRIED CAJUN SALMON

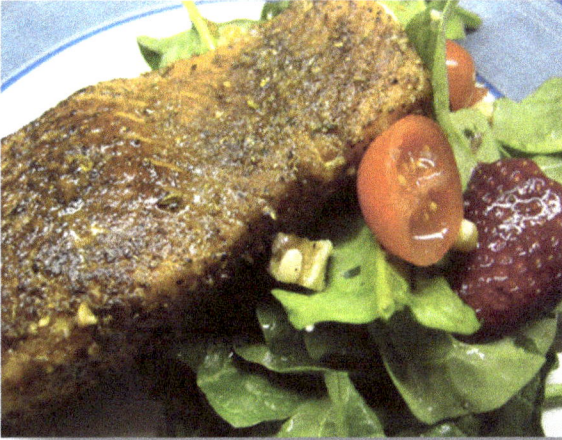

Preparation Time: 9 minutes

Cooking Time: 10 minutes

Servings: 1

Nutritional values:

- Calories: 216 kcal
- Fat: 19 g
- Carbohydrates: 5.6g
- Proteins: 19.2 g

Ingredients:

- 1 piece fresh salmon
- 2 tbsp. Cajun seasoning
- Lemon juice.

Directions:

1. Let the air fryer preheat to 180°C.
2. Pat dry the salmon fillet. Rub lemon juice and Cajun seasoning over the fish fillet.
3. Place in the air fryer, cook for 7 minutes. Serve with salad greens and lime wedges.

BUFFALO CHICKEN HOT WINGS

Preparation Time: 10 minutes

Cooking Time: 20-25 minutes

Servings: 6

Nutritional values:

- Calories: 88
- Fat: 6.5 g
- Carbohydrates: 2.6 g
- Proteins: 4.5 g

Ingredients:

- 16 chicken wings, pastured
- 1 tsp. garlic powder
- 2 tsp. chicken seasoning
- ¾ tsp. ground black pepper

- 2 tsp. soy sauce

- ¼ cup buffalo sauce, reduced-fat

Directions:

1. Switch on the air fryer, insert fryer basket, grease it with olive oil, then shut with its lid, set the fryer at 400°F and preheat for 5 minutes.

2. Meanwhile, place chicken wings in a bowl, drizzle with soy sauce, toss until well coated, and then, season with black pepper and garlic powder.

3. Open the fryer, stack chicken wings in it, then spray with oil and close with its lid.

4. Cook the chicken wings for 10 minutes, turning the wings halfway through, and then transfer them to a bowl, covering the bowl with a foil to keep the chicken wings warm.

5. Air fry the remaining chicken wings in the same manner, then transfer them to the bowl, add buffalo sauce and toss until well coated.

6. Return chicken wings into the fryer basket in a single layer and continue frying for 7 to 12 minutes or until chicken wings are glazed and crispy, shaking the chicken wings every 3 to 4 minutes.

7. Serve straight away.

CHICKEN WITH CASHEW NUTS

Preparation Time: 10 minutes

Cooking Time: 10-15 minutes

Servings: 4

Nutritional values:

- Calories: 425 kcal
- Fat: 35 g
- Carbohydrates: 25 g
- Proteins: 53 g

Ingredients:

- 1 lb. chicken cubes
- 2 tbsp. soy sauce
- 1 tbsp. corn flour
- 2 ½ onion cubes
- 1 carrot, chopped
- 1/3 cup cashew nuts, fried

- 1 capsicum, cut
- 2 tbsp. garlic, crushed
- Salt and white pepper

Directions:

1. Marinate the chicken cubes with ½ tbsp. of white pepper, ½ tsp. salt, 2 tbsp. soya sauce, and add 1 tbsp. corn flour.

2. Set aside for 25 minutes. Preheat the Air Fryer to 380°F and transfer the marinated chicken. Add the garlic, the onion, the capsicum, and the carrot; fry for 5–6 minutes. Roll it in the cashew nuts before serving.

FRIED CHICKEN TAMARI AND MUSTARD

Preparation Time: 10 minutes

Cooking Time: 30 minutes

Servings: 4

Nutritional values:

- Calories: 100 kcal
- Fat: 6 g
- Carbohydrates: 0 g
- Proteins: 18 g

Ingredients:

- 1kg very small chopped chicken
- Tamari Sauce
- Original mustard
- Ground pepper
- 1 lemon

- Flour
- Extra virgin olive oil

Directions:

1. Put the chicken in a bowl; you can put the chicken with or without the skin to everyone's taste.
2. Add a generous stream of tamari, one or two tbsp. of mustard, a little ground pepper, and a splash of lemon juice.
3. Link everything very well and let macerate for an hour.
4. Pass the chicken pieces for flour and place them in the air fryer basket.
5. Put 20 minutes at 200°C. At halftime, move the chicken from the basket.
6. Do not crush the chicken; it is preferable to make two or three batches of chicken to pile up and do not fry the pieces well.

HERBED CHICKEN

Preparation Time: 10 minutes

Cooking Time: 40 minutes

Servings: 4

Nutritional values:

- Calories: 390 kcal
- Fat: 10 g
- Carbohydrates: 22 g
- Proteins: 20 g

Ingredients:

- 1 whole chicken
- 1 tsp. garlic powder
- 1 tsp. onion powder
- ½ tsp. thyme; dried
- 1 tsp. rosemary; dried
- 1 tbsp. lemon juice
- 2 tbsp. olive oil
- Salt and black pepper to the taste

Directions:

1. Season chicken with salt and pepper, rub with thyme, rosemary, garlic powder, and onion powder, rub with lemon juice and olive oil and leave aside for 30 minutes.

2. Put the chicken in your air fryer and cook at 360°F for 20 minutes on each side. Leave chicken aside to cool down, carve and serve.

SALTED BISCUIT PIE TURKEY CHOPS

Preparation Time: 10 minutes

Cooking Time: 30 minutes

Servings: 4

Nutritional values:

- Calories: 126 kcal
- Fat: 6 g
- Carbohydrates: 0 g
- Proteins: 18 g

Ingredients:

- 8 large turkey chops
- 300 gr crackers
- 2 eggs
- Extra virgin olive oil
- Salt
- Ground pepper

Directions:

1. Put the turkey chops on the worktable, and salt and pepper.
2. Beat the eggs in a bowl.
3. Crush the cookies in the Thermo mix with a few turbo strokes until they are made grit, or you can crush them with the blender.
4. Put the cookies in a bowl.
5. Pass the chops through the beaten egg and then passed them through the crushed cookies. Press well so that the empanada is perfect.
6. Paint the empanada with a silicone brush and extra virgin olive oil.
7. Put the chops in the basket of the air fryer; not all will enter. They will be done in batches.
8. Select 200°C and 15 minutes.
9. When you have all the chops made, serve.

CREAMY CHICKEN, PEAS AND RICE

Preparation Time: 10 minutes

Cooking Time: 30 minutes

Servings: 4

Nutritional values:

- Calories: 313 kcal
- Fat: 12 g
- Carbohydrates: 27 g
- Proteins: 44 g

Ingredients:

- 1 lb. chicken breasts; skinless, boneless, and cut into quarters
- 1 cup white rice; already cooked
- 1 cup chicken stock
- ¼ cup parsley; chopped.
- 2 cups peas; frozen

- 1 ½ cups parmesan; grated
- 1 tbsp. olive oil
- 3 garlic cloves; minced
- 1 yellow onion; chopped
- ½ cup white wine
- ¼ cup heavy cream
- Salt and black pepper to the taste

Directions:

1. Season chicken breasts with salt and pepper, drizzle half of the oil over them, rub well, put in your air fryer's basket, and cook them at 360|F for 6 minutes.

2. Preheat the pan with the rest of the oil over medium-high heat, add garlic, onion, and wine, stock, salt, pepper, and heavy cream; stir and simmer. Cook for 9 minutes.

3. Transfer chicken breasts into a heatproof dish that fits your air fryer, add peas, rice, and cream mix over them, toss, and sprinkle parmesan and parsley all over, place in your air fryer and cook at 420|F for 10 minutes. Divide among plates and serve hot.

CHINESE STUFFED CHICKEN

Preparation Time: 10 minutes

Cooking Time: 35-40 minutes

Servings: 8

Nutritional values:

- Calories: 320 kcal
- Fat: 12 g
- Carbohydrates: 22 g
- Proteins: 12 g

Ingredients:

- 1 whole chicken
- 10 wolfberries
- 2 red chilies; chopped
- 4 ginger slices
- 1 yam; cubed
- 1 tsp. soy sauce
- 3 tsp. sesame oil
- Salt and white pepper to the taste

Directions:

1. Season chicken with salt, pepper, rub with soy sauce and sesame oil, and stuff with wolfberries, yam cubes, chilies, and ginger.
2. Place in your air fryer, cook at 400°F for 20 minutes, and then, at 360 F for 15 minutes. Carve chicken, divide among plates, and serve.

ROASTED VEGGIES

Preparation Time: 6 minutes

Cooking Time: 15 minutes

Servings: 4

Nutritional values:

- Calories: 35 kcal
- Fat: 2.6 g
- Carbohydrates: 3.3 g
- Proteins: 1.3 g

Ingredients:

- ½ cup each
- Summer squash (diced)
- Zucchini (diced)
- Mushrooms (diced)
- Cauliflower (diced)
- Asparagus (diced)

- Sweet red pepper (diced)
- 2 tsps. vegetable oil
- ¼ tsp. salt
- ½ tsp. black pepper (ground)
- 1 tsp. seasoning

Directions:

1. Preheat air fryer at 180°C.
2. Mix all the veggies, oil, pepper, seasoning, and salt in a bowl. Toss well for coating.
3. Cook the mixture of veggies in the air fryer for ten minutes.

TEMPURA VEGETABLES

Preparation Time: 9 minutes

Cooking Time: 10-15 minutes

Servings: 4

Nutritional values:

- Calories: 242
- Fat: 9.3 g
- Carbohydrates: 35.6 g
- Proteins: 9.2 g

Ingredients:

Half cup each:

- Flour
- Green beans
- Onion rings
- Asparagus spears
- Sweet pepper rings
- Zucchini slices
- Avocado wedges

- ½ tsp. each
- Black pepper (ground)
- Salt
- 2 large eggs
- 2 tbsp. water
- 1 cup panko bread crumbs
- 2 tsps. vegetable oil

Directions:

1. Combine flour, pepper, and one-fourth tsp. of salt in a dish.
2. Combine water and eggs in a shallow dish.
3. Mix oil and bread crumbs in another shallow dish.
4. Sprinkle remaining salt over the veggies.
5. Dip the veggies in the mixture of flour, then in the mixture of egg, and then coat in bread crumbs.
6. Cook the veggies in the air fryer for ten minutes. Shake in between.

EGGPLANT PARMESAN

Preparation Time: 5 minutes

Cooking Time: 32 minutes

Servings: 4

Nutritional values:

- Calories: 370 kcal
- Fat: 17 g
- Carbohydrates: 35.6 g
- Proteins: 24 g

Ingredients:

- ½ cup bread crumbs (Italian)
- ¼ cup parmesan cheese (grated)
- 1 tsp. each
- Salt
- Italian seasoning
- ½ tsp. each
- Basil (dried)
- Garlic powder

- Onion powder
- Black pepper (ground)
- 1 cup flour
- 2 large eggs (beaten)
- 1 eggplant (sliced in a round of half an inch)
- 1/3 cup marinara sauce
- 8 slices mozzarella cheese

Directions:

1. Mix parmesan cheese, bread crumbs, seasoning, basil, salt, onion powder, garlic powder, and black pepper together in a mixing bowl.
2. Add flour in a shallow dish.
3. Beat the eggs in a bowl.
4. Dip the slices of eggplants in flour and then in eggs. Coat the eggplants in the mixture of bread crumbs.
5. Cook the eggplants in the air fryer for ten minutes. Flip and cook for four minutes.
6. Top the slices of eggplants with one slice of mozzarella cheese and marinara sauce.
7. Cook again for two minutes.
8. Serve hot.

FRENCH FRIES

Preparation Time: 6 minutes

Cooking Time: 20-25 minutes

Servings: 4

Nutritional values:

- Calories: 108 kcal
- Fat: 2.1 g
- Carbohydrates: 17.9 g
- Proteins: 2.4 g

Ingredients:

- 1 pound of russet potatoes (peeled)
- 2 tsps. vegetable oil
- 1 pinch cayenne pepper
- ½ tsp. salt

Directions:

1. Cut the potatoes in half-inch slices lengthwise.
2. Soak the potatoes in water for five minutes.
3. Drain the water and soak again in boiling water for ten minutes.
4. Drain all the water. Pat dry using paper towels.
5. Add oil and cayenne pepper. Season with salt.
6. Cook the potatoes for fifteen minutes. Toss with some salt and cook again for five minutes.

SWEET AND SPICY CARROTS

Preparation Time: 9 minutes

Cooking Time: 24 minutes

Servings: 2

Nutritional values:

- Calories: 128 kcal
- Fat: 6 g
- Carbohydrates: 17.2 g
- Proteins: 1.2 g

Ingredients:

- 1 serving cooking spray
- 1 tbsp. each
- Hot honey
- Butter (melted)
- Orange zest
- Orange juice
- ½ tsp. cardamom (ground)

- ½ pound baby carrots
- 1/3 tsp. black pepper and salt

Directions:

1. Heat your air fryer at 200°C. Use a cooking spray for greasing the basket.
2. Mix honey, butter, cardamom, and orange zest in a small bowl.
3. Pour the sauce over the carrots and coat well.
4. Cook the carrots for twenty minutes. Toss in between.
5. Mix orange juice with the leftover sauce.
6. Serve the carrots with sauce from the top.

AIR FRIED POTATOES

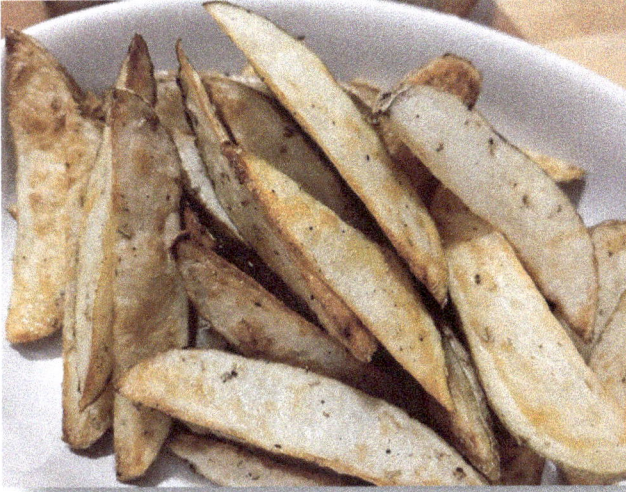

Preparation Time: 7 minutes

Cooking Time: 62 minutes

Servings: 2

Nutritional values:

- Calories: 310 kcal
- Fat: 6.3 g
- Carbohydrates: 61.5 g
- Proteins: 7.2 g

Ingredients:

- 2 large potatoes
- 1 tbsp. peanut oil
- ½ tsp. sea salt

Directions:

1. Heat your air fryer at 200°C.
2. Brush the potatoes with oil. Sprinkle some salt.
3. Place the potatoes in the basket of the air fryer and cook for one hour.
4. Serve hot by dividing the potatoes from the center.

ASPARAGUS AVOCADO SOUP

Preparation Time: 9 minutes

Cooking Time: 22 minutes

Servings: 4

Nutritional values:

- Calories: 208 kcal
- Fat: 11 g
- Carbohydrates: 2 g
- Proteins: 4 g

Ingredients:

- 1 avocado, peeled, pitted, cubed
- 12 ounces asparagus
- ½-tsp. ground black pepper
- 1-tsp. garlic powder
- 1-tsp. sea salt
- 2 tbsp. olive oil, divided
- ½ lemon, juiced
- 2 cups vegetable stock

Directions:

1. Switch on the air fryer, insert fryer basket, grease it with olive oil, then shut with its lid, set the fryer at 425°F and preheat for 5 minutes.

2. Meanwhile, place asparagus in a shallow dish, drizzle with 1-tbsp. oil, sprinkle with garlic powder, salt, and black pepper, and toss until well mixed.

3. Open the fryer, add asparagus in it, close with its lid and cook for 10 minutes until nicely golden and roasted, shaking halfway through the frying.

4. When the air fryer beeps, open its lid and transfer asparagus to a food processor.

5. Add remaining ingredients into a food processor and pulse until well combined and smooth.

6. Tip the soup in a saucepan, pour in water if the soup is too thick, and heat it over medium-low heat for 5 minutes until thoroughly heated.

7. Ladle soup into bowls and serve.

ROASTED POTATOES

Preparation Time: 11 minutes

Cooking Time: 23 minutes

Servings: 4

Nutritional values:

- Calories: 93
- Fat: 0.2 g
- Carbohydrates: 9 g
- Proteins: 1 g

Ingredients:

- 227 g small fresh potatoes, cleaned and halved
- 30 ml olive oil
- 3 g salt
- 1 g black pepper
- 2 g garlic powder
- 1 g dried thyme
- 1 g dried rosemary

Directions:

1. Preheat the air fryer for a few minutes. Set it to 195°C.

2. Cover the potatoes in half with olive oil and mix the seasonings.

3. Place the potatoes in the preheated air fryer. Set the time to 20 minutes. Be sure to shake the baskets in the middle of cooking.

HONEY ROASTED CARROTS

Preparation Time: 9 minutes

Cooking Time: 13 minutes

Servings: 4

Nutritional values:

- Calories: 123 kcal
- Fat: 42 g
- Carbohydrates: 9 g
- Proteins: 1 g

Ingredients:

- 454 g rainbow carrots, peeled and washed
- 15 ml olive oil
- 30 ml honey
- 2 sprigs fresh thyme
- Salt and pepper to taste

Directions:

1. Wash the carrots and dry them with a paper towel. Leave aside.
2. Preheat the air fryer for a few minutes at 180°C.
3. Place the carrots in a bowl with olive oil, honey, thyme, salt, and pepper. Place the carrots in the air fryer at 180°C for 12 minutes. Be sure to shake the baskets in the middle of cooking.

SUGAR-FREE AIR FRIED CARROT CAKE

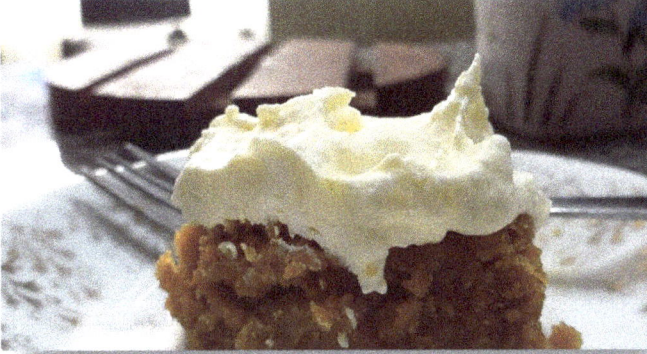

Preparation Time: 14 minutes

Cooking Time: 41 minutes

Servings: 8

Nutritional values:

- Calories 287 kcal
- Fat: 22 g
- Carbohydrates: 19 g
- Proteins: 4 g

Ingredients:

- 1 ¼ cups all-purpose flour
- 1 tsp. pumpkin pie spice
- one tsp. baking powder
- 3/4 cup Splenda
- 2 cups carrots–grated
- 2 eggs
- 1/2 tsp. baking soda
- ¾ cup canola oil

Directions:

1. Let the air fryer preheat to 350°F. Spray the cake pan with oil spray.
2. And add flour over that.
3. In a bowl, combine the baking powder, flour, pumpkin pie spice, and baking soda.
4. In another bowl, mix the eggs, oil, and sugar alternative. Now combine the dry to wet ingredients.
5. Add half of the dry ingredients first mix and the other half of the dry mixture.
6. Add in the grated carrots.
7. Add the cake batter to the greased cake pan.
8. Place the cake pan in the basket of the air fryer.

9. Let it Air fry for half an hour, but do not let the top too brown.

10. If the top is browning, add a piece of foil over the top of the cake.

11. Air fry it until a toothpick comes out clean, 35–40 minutes in total.

12. Let the cake cool down before serving.

SUGAR-FREE LOW CARB CHEESECAKE MUFFINS

Preparation Time: 16 minutes

Cooking Time: 28 minutes

Servings: 18

Nutritional values:

- Calories: 93 kcal
- Fat: 9 g
- Carbohydrates: 1 g
- Proteins: 2 g

Ingredients:

- 1/2 cup Splenda
- 1 ½ cup cream cheese
- 2 eggs
- 1 tsp. vanilla extract

Directions:

1. Let the oven preheat to 300°F.

2. Spray the muffin pan with oil.

3. In a bowl, add the sugar alternative, vanilla extract, and cream cheese. Mix well

4. Add-in the eggs gently, one at a time. Do not over mix the batter.

5. Let it bake for 25 to 30 minutes or until cooked.

6. Take out from the air fryer and let them cool before adding frosting.

7. Serve and enjoy.

SUGAR-FREE AIR FRIED CHOCOLATE DONUT HOLES

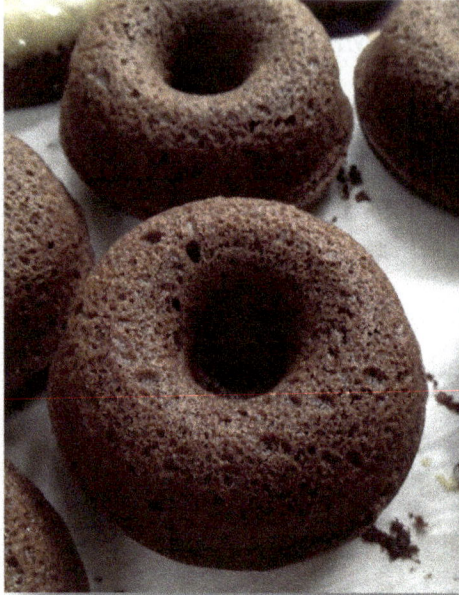

Preparation Time: 15 minutes

Cooking Time: 16 minutes

Servings: 32

Nutritional values:

- Calories 22 kcal
- Fat: 2 g

- Carbohydrates: 1 g
- Proteins: 1 g

Ingredients:

- 6 tbsp. Splenda
- 1 cup any flour
- 1/2 tsp. baking soda
- 6 tbsp. unsweetened cocoa powder
- 3 tbsp. butter
- 1 egg
- 1/2 tsp. baking powder
- 2 tbsp. unsweetened chocolate chopped
- ¼ cup plain yogurt

Directions:

1. In a big mixing bowl, combine the baking powder, baking soda, and flour.
2. Then add in the cocoa powder and sugar alternative.
3. In a mug or microwave-safe bowl, melt the butter and the unsweetened chocolate.
4. Mix every 15 seconds and make sure they melt together and combine well.
5. Set it aside to cool it down.

6. In that big mixing bowl from before, add in the yogurt and the egg. Add in the melted butter and chocolate mixture. Cover the bowl with plastic wrap and let it chill in the refrigerator for 30 minutes.

7. To make the donut balls, take out the batter from the fridge.

8. With the help of a tbsp., scoop out sufficient batter so a donut ball will form with your hands.

9. You can use oil on your hands if the dough is too sticky.

10. Spray the oil on the air fryer basket and sprinkle with flour and let it preheat to 350°F.

11. Work in batches and add the balls in one single layer.

12. Let it bake for 10–12 minutes until they are done. To check doneness, try a toothpick if it comes out clean.

13. Take out from air fryer, let it cool and serve hot or cold.

SUGAR-FREE LOW CARB PEANUT BUTTER COOKIES

Preparation Time: 16 minutes

Cooking Time: 8-10 minutes

Servings: 23

Nutritional values:

- Calories: 198 kcal
- Carbohydrates: 7 g
- Proteins: 9 g
- Fat: 17 g

Ingredients:

- 1 cup all-natural 100% peanut butter
- 1 whisked egg
- 1 tsp. liquid stevia drops
- 1 cup sugar alternative

Directions:

1. Mix all the ingredients into a dough. Make 24 balls with your hands from the combined dough.

2. On a cookie sheet or cutting board, press the dough balls with the help of a fork to form a crisscross pattern.

3. Add six cookies to the basket of the air fryer in a single layer. Make sure the cookies are separated from each other. Cook in batches

4. Let them Air Fry, for 8–10 minutes, at 325°F. Take the basket out from the air fryer.

5. Let the cookies cool for one minute, then with care, take the cookies out.

6. Keep baking the rest of the peanut butter cookies in batches.

7. Let them cool completely and serve.

AIR FRYER BLUEBERRY MUFFINS

Preparation Time: 9 minutes

Cooking Time: 16 minutes

Servings: 8

Nutritional values:

- Calories: 213 kcal
- Fat: 10 g
- Carbohydrates: 13.2 g
- Proteins: 9.7 g

Ingredients:

- ½ cup sugar alternative
- 1 and 1/3 cup flour
- 1/3 cup oil
- 2 tsp. of baking powder
- ¼ tsp. salt
- 1 egg

- ½ cup milk
- 8 muffin cups (foil) with paper liners
- Or silicone baking cups
- 2/3 cup frozen and thawed blueberries or fresh

Directions:

1. Let the air fryer preheat to 330°F.
2. In a large bowl, sift together baking powder, salt, sugar, and flour. Mix well
3. In another bowl, add milk, oil, and egg mix it well.
4. To the dry ingredients to the egg mix, mix until combined but do not over mix
5. Add the blueberries carefully. Pour the mixture into muffin paper cups or muffin baking tray
6. Put four muffin cups in the air fryer basket or add more if your basket's size is big.
7. Cook for 12–14 minutes, at 330°F, or until when touch lightly the tops, it should spring back.
8. Cook the remaining muffins accordingly.
9. Take out from the air fryer and let them cool before serving.

www.ingramcontent.com/pod-product-compliance
Lightning Source LLC
Chambersburg PA
CBHW050745030426
42336CB00012B/1670